Therapeutic Exercise for Athletic Injuries Lab Manual

ATHLETIC TRAINING EDUCATION SERIES

LINDA S. LEVY, MEd, ATC and JULIE N. BERNIER, EdD, ATC
PLYMOUTH STATE COLLEGE

DAVID H. PERRIN, PhD, ATC
SERIES EDITOR
UNIVERSITY OF VIRGINIA, CHARLOTTESVILLE

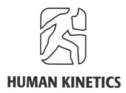

HUMAN KINETICS

ISBN: 0-7360-3382-3

Acquisitions Editor: Loarn D. Robertson, PhD
Developmental Editor: Joanna Hatzopoulos
Managing Editor: Susan C. Hagan
Copyeditor: Joyce Sexton
Proofreader: Coree Schutter
Graphic Designer: Stuart Cartwright
Graphic Artist: Angela K. Snyder
Cover Designer: Stuart Cartwright
Art Manager: Craig Newsom
Mac Artist: Angela K. Snyder
Printer: Versa Press

Printed in the United States of America
10 9 8 7 6 5 4 3 2 1

Human Kinetics
Web site: www.humankinetics.com

United States: Human Kinetics
P.O. Box 5076
Champaign, IL 61825-5076
800-747-4457
e-mail: humank@hkusa.com

Canada: Human Kinetics
475 Devonshire Road Unit 100
Windsor, ON N8Y 2L5
800-465-7301 (in Canada only)
e-mail: hkcan@mnsi.net

Europe: Human Kinetics
P.O. Box IW14
Leeds LS16 6TR, United Kingdom
+44 (0) 113 278 1708
e-mail: humank@hkeurope.com

Australia: Human Kinetics
57A Price Avenue
Lower Mitcham, South Australia 5062
08 8277 1555
e-mail: liahka@senet.com.au

New Zealand: Human Kinetics
P.O. Box 105-231, Auckland Central
09-523-3462
e-mail: hkp@ihug.co.nz

This lab manual is dedicated to our students, past and present. They were willing to be our guinea pigs as we developed these labs. Their critique and words of encouragement equaled their excitement and enthusiasm. Thanks to all of them.

CONTENTS

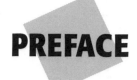

PREFACE

This lab manual was written to accompany the Athletic Training Education Series textbook *Therapeutic Exercise for Athletic Injuries.* There is not a lab for every chapter in the text; rather, the labs included in this manual reflect specific applications in therapeutic exercise that you need to be able to perform to work in a clinical setting.

The certified athletic trainer must have particular skills to become a therapeutic exercise clinician. Those skills are based on knowing how the various forms of open and closed kinetic chain therapeutic exercises affect the healing process. This lab manual is designed to help you acquire that knowledge.

As you learn didactic information from the textbook, you can use the lab manual as a vehicle for applying those concepts and ideas. Although most labs can be completed in 1 to 1+ hours, you may need additional time to fully explore, and become proficient at, each lab's content.

A quick review of the table of contents will reveal that this lab manual does not specifically include detailed therapeutic exercise protocols for all injuries. Instead, the last three labs are dedicated to exercises applicable to injuries of the trunk and the upper and lower extremities. You obtain an idea of potential exercises that can be prescribed and then select which exercises to include, depending on the nature and severity of the injury.

Instructor's note: *Answers to the lab activities are provided in the* Therapeutic Exercise for Athletic Injuries Instructor Guide.

LAB 1

Mechanical Concepts

The purpose of this lab is to reinforce mechanical concepts related to rehabilitation by providing you with experiences in rehabilitation that incorporate the concepts of lever types, torque, active/passive insufficiency, effect of segmental stabilization, and effect of gravity.

Review material from chapter 3 of the textbook before completing this lab.

OBJECTIVES

- You should distinguish between first-, second-, and third-class levers as related to machines and the human body, and cite the advantages and disadvantages of each.

- You should understand how changes in lever arm affect torque.

- You should be able to explain and demonstrate the effects of active and passive insufficiency of two-joint muscles.

Name_____ Date_____

Activities

1. **Levers.** In the following tables, describe each of the types of levers. Give one example of a machine or device and one example in the body for each type of lever.

First Class

Description	Machine/device	Lever arrangement in the body

Second Class

Description	Machine/device	Lever arrangement in the body

Third Class

Description	Machine/device	Lever arrangement in the body

A. What is the advantage of each type of lever arrangement?
- First class

- Second class

- Third class

B. Which type of lever arrangement predominates in the body?

C. What is the consequence of this?

2. **Torque.** After reviewing the concept of torque, perform this lab activity and answer the questions that follow.

Equipment needed: *broomstick handle (cut to 3 ft [.9 m]), 5-lb weight, athletic tape, tape measure or ruler. Place enough tape around one end of the handle to hold the weight in place. Slide the weight onto the handle from the opposite end. Secure the weight at the end with another row of tape. Measure from the weight and place a mark every 6 in. (15 cm).*

A. Grasp the handle with the weight on your thumb side as close to the weight as possible. Stand upright with arm at your side. Keeping your elbow fully extended and shoulder still, perform radial deviation of the wrist against the resistance of the weight. Now move your hand to the first line (6-in. mark) and repeat. Repeat this action at each marker. Note the increased difficulty as you move away from the weight.

B. Define the following terms:
- Torque

- Lever arm

- Force

C. Answer the following questions:

1. How can you use the information you have gained from this lab when performing manual muscle tests?

2. How can you use the information you have gained from this lab to make it easier for the patient when performing a manual muscle test or resistance exercise?

3. How can you use this information to make it easier for you?

4. During this lab, where was the axis of rotation (fulcrum) during this action?

5. Where is the resistance?

6. Where is the force?

7. What type of lever system is this?

8. With your hand at the 6-in. mark, how much torque **does the weight** produce when you hold the weight level with the floor?

9. At the 1-ft mark?

10. At 1.5 ft?

11. At 2 ft?

12. How much torque **must you produce** to hold the weight horizontal when you are holding the handle at the 1-ft mark?

13. For illustrative purposes, let's assume that the lever arm for the muscular force is 1 in. How much force must you generate in order to produce the required torque to hold the handle horizontal when your hand is 12 in. from the weight? In other words, how much muscular force does it take to hold the 5-lb weight when your hand is 12 in. from the weight?

14. How can you use the information you have gained from this lab when having patients perform resistance exercises?

3. **Active and passive insufficiency.** After reviewing the concept of active and passive insufficiency, answer the questions that follow and perform the lab activity.

Equipment needed: *This lab is designed to be completed with or without a handheld dynamometer. If a dynamometer is available, assess muscle performance using the dynamometer; if not, follow the same instructions using manual muscle testing.*

A. Answer the following questions:

1. How much is a muscle capable of shortening (in percentage terms)?

2. How does the fact that a muscle is a two-joint muscle affect its ability to shorten?

3. Active insufficiency occurs when a muscle is called upon to shorten over both joints. Give one example in the lower extremity, one in the upper extremity, and one in the spine of a situation in which active insufficiency will hinder performance.

   - Lower

   - Upper

   - Spine

B. **Rectus femoris lab.** The rectus femoris muscle is a two-joint muscle contributing to hip flexion and knee extension. A muscle is capable of shortening only so far. When the muscle is called upon to shorten over both of its joints (i.e., to perform hip flexion and knee extension simultaneously), it cannot do so with its normal strength. Test this theory by performing a manual muscle test of the quadriceps muscles in two different positions, once with the hip extended and once with the hip flexed, according to the following instructions.

Have your partner sit on a table with knee and hip flexed to 90°. Have your partner extend his/her knee. When the knee is almost fully extended (last 25°), assess strength either with a handheld dynamometer or manually. Apply the force just above the ankle joint. Your partner may hold on to the edge of the table for support.

Perform the same test, but this time have your partner lie supine at the edge of the table. Again assess knee extension in the last 25°.

1. In which position did your partner exert more force?

2. Ask your partner which position felt more advantageous.

4. **Stabilization.** For each of the actions listed, name the muscles (or muscle groups) and any special considerations (e.g., two-joint muscles or muscles that contribute only in a certain position; substitute motions to watch out for). With this information, experiment in finding the optimal position for performing a manual muscle test. Be sure to stabilize proximal joints, and do not allow substitute motions. Finally, describe the optimal test position.

Shoulder Abduction

Muscles	Special considerations	Optimal test position

Shoulder External Rotation

Muscles	Special considerations	Optimal test position

Elbow Flexion

Muscles	Special considerations	Optimal test position

Wrist Extension

Muscles	Special considerations	Optimal test position

5. **Gravity.** Perform the tests described and answer the questions that follow.

> A. Perform a manual muscle test of the middle deltoid muscle. Assume that the person can perform to grade 4-5. Compare bilaterally.

How did you perform this test?

> B. Perform a manual muscle test of the hip flexors. Assume that the person can perform to grade 4-5.

How did you perform this test?

> C. Now assume that your patient cannot perform this motion through full active ROM against gravity. Perform a manual muscle test of this same muscle (muscle group) in such a way that gravity will not have any effect on the motion.

Describe how you did this test for the middle deltoid and for the hip flexors.

LAB 2

Rehabilitation Assessment

The purpose of this lab is to encourage you to think critically about the assessment results before initiating a rehabilitation program, and to apply those results to a SOAP note.

Review material from chapter 4 of the textbook before completing this lab.

OBJECTIVES

- You should distinguish between an initial injury assessment and follow-up assessments necessary for safe, effective rehabilitation progressions.

- You should know how to record your assessment findings.

Name_____ Date_____

Activities

1. For each case study, perform an assessment to determine each patient's treatment plan.

   Case A. Two days after Carol sustained a grade II ankle sprain, she is beginning her rehabilitation program. Before you begin rehabilitation, you must reassess her injury.

   1. What will you include?

   2. What will you leave out?

   3. What will be your treatment plan for the day?

   4. What will you do to assess the effectiveness of your treatment?

   Case B. Jason is an injured lacrosse player with biceps tendinitis. During your initial assessment, you were unable to determine his full shoulder strength because of his pain. You would like to begin a shoulder rehab program, but are unsure where to begin. Reassess his situation now that he has rested his arm for one week.

   1. What strength tests will you perform?

   2. What should you expect to find?

   3. What rehab tools that improve strength are available to you?

4. What exercises will you begin with?

5. How will you know if they are effective or if you've prescribed too much?

Case C. You have been treating a hamstring strain during a diver's pre-season. It is now 1.5 weeks into the rehab program and you want to know if he is responding to your choice of treatments. Reassess the hamstring strain.

1. What tests will you perform?

2. How will you know if your treatment protocol is effective?

3. What functional activities can you prescribe?

2. Develop a SOAP note using the following case study.

Case Study. Your orthopedic team physician has diagnosed a patient with a second-degree right wrist sprain. Through questioning you have found the following:

- The patient is a 19-year-old male ice hockey player.
- An incident in which he was forced into the boards caused his wrist to hyperextend.
- He complains of pain on anterior, distal ulna.
- He complains of pain on distal ulna with ulnar deviation and circumduction.
- All complaints of pain are graded II on I–IV scale.
- There is no previous history related to this injury.
- The patient drives to school.
- He owns a car with a stick shift.
- He is eager to return to practice and competition.

From the objective tests you performed, you found the following:

- (+) Swelling
- (–) Discoloration
- (–) Deformity
- (+) Pain on anterior/distal ulna
- (+) Pain with wrist distraction
- (+) Pain with wrist flexion
- (+) Pain with AROM in ulnar deviation
- (+) Pain with AROM and PROM in extension
- (+) Tap test in wrist extension

LAB 3

Goniometry

The purpose of this lab is to challenge you to become proficient at using a goniometer.

Review material from chapter 5 of the textbook before completing this lab.

OBJECTIVES

- You should understand the average ranges of motion for joints in both the upper and lower extremities.

- You should understand proper goniometer alignment.

- You should be familiar with the use of all sizes of goniometers.

- You should measure joint angles.

- You should describe joint position relative to joint angle.

Name_____   Date_____

Activities

1. Demonstrate the use of a goniometer by measuring active and passive ROM for the joint angles listed. Select a partner. Your partner should move through his or her minimum and maximum ranges of motion in both gravity-dependent and gravity-eliminated positions when applicable.

Equipment needed: *15-cm (6-in.) goniometer, smaller goniometer for measuring ankle and wrist joints*

Use a partner and a goniometer for each of the following problems. Find the minimum and maximum ranges for each motion.

A. Gravity-dependent active knee flexion
- Trial 1
- Trial 2
- Trial 3

B. Active ankle dorsi- and plantar flexion
- Trial 1
- Trial 2
- Trial 3

C. Passive ankle dorsi- and plantar flexion
- Trial 1
- Trial 2
- Trial 3

D. Active wrist extension
- Trial 1
- Trial 2
- Trial 3

E. Gravity-dependent active shoulder flexion
- Trial 1
- Trial 2
- Trial 3

F. Gravity-eliminated active shoulder flexion
- Trial 1
- Trial 2
- Trial 3

G. Gravity-dependent active shoulder external rotation
- Trial 1
- Trial 2
- Trial 3

H. Gravity-eliminated passive shoulder external rotation
- Trial 1
- Trial 2
- Trial 3

I. Active lumbar extension
- Trial 1
- Trial 2
- Trial 3

J. In B (active ankle dorsi- and plantar flexion), where is 0°?
- Trial 1
- Trial 2
- Trial 3

2. For each of the following situations, estimate the ROM that would be available for each condition.

A. What would you expect the knee ROM to be for an athlete who has no terminal extension due to swelling?

B. How much motion is possible in hip extension if the rectus femoris has sustained a second-degree strain?

C. How much motion is possible when the elbow is taped for a hyperextension injury?

3. Describe joint position by placing the joint at the pre-set ROM listed.

A. What position would an athlete be in when his/her _____ joint is at _____ degrees?

B. Ankle joint is at 110°

C. GH joint is at 165°

D. Knee joint is at 155°

E. MCP joint is at 30°, the PIP joint is at 60°, and the DIP joint is at 30°

LAB 4

Massage

The purpose of this lab is to provide you with practice in performing massage and to enable you to incorporate massage into a therapeutic rehabilitation program.

Review material from chapter 6 of the textbook before completing this lab.

OBJECTIVES

- You should demonstrate proper hygiene before performing massage.

- You should understand indications and contraindications for massage.

- You should demonstrate patient draping and positioning for massage to various body parts.

- You should explain massage cautions to the patient.

- You should explain the use of massage lubricants.

- You should explain and demonstrate the massage techniques of effleurage, petrissage, and friction.

Name_____ Date_____

Activities

For each of the following case studies, perform leg, arm, low back, shoulder, and neck massage on a partner utilizing the massage techniques appropriate to each case study. Change partners for every case study. Demonstrate proper stroke technique, adhere to proper hygiene, apply appropriate patient positioning and draping, explain massage cautions, and use the appropriate lubricants.

Case A. Bill is an 18-year-old male trying out for the men's downhill ski team. After one week of intensive preseason training that includes plyometrics and hill running, he limps into the athletic training room complaining of gastroc spasms. You decide that in addition to ice, stretching, and rehydration, massage may help relieve his cramping. Perform a leg massage on your partner as if he/she had presented with these signs and symptoms.

Case B. John is a 35-year-old "weekend" athlete. Two days after his first ice hockey game of the season, he complains of muscle soreness in his right triceps, his dominant side. After a thorough evaluation, you determine that he is experiencing delayed-onset muscle soreness. Following stretching exercises, you decide to try massage. Perform an upper arm massage on your partner as if he/she had presented with these signs and symptoms.

Case C. Kate is a second-string soccer goalie who has been diagnosed with chronic low back spasms. Today she is going through a particularly hard practice that requires her to retrieve many ground balls. Halfway through practice you notice that she is getting up slowly, finally coming over to let you know that her low back is in spasm. Perform a low back massage on your partner—one that can be used on the field.

Case D. Sally is a rugby player who got tackled going for a loose ball. The tackle caused her to roll over her left shoulder with her head laterally flexed to her right. Now she complains of pain in her left upper traps. You decide that an e-stim treatment followed by massage would help. Perform a shoulder and neck massage on your partner as if he/she had presented with these signs and symptoms.

Case E. Mark is a 25-year-old computer specialist at the company where you work as an athletic trainer. He has been referred to you because of his hamstring muscle pain. He tells you that he has been jogging during lunch hours and has recently increased his mileage. Part of the rehabilitation program that you design includes massage. Perform a hamstring massage on your partner as if he/she had presented with these signs and symptoms.

LAB 5

Joint Mobilization

The purpose of this lab is to teach you how to apply joint mobilization techniques.

Review material from chapter 6 of the textbook before completing this lab.

OBJECTIVES

- You should understand fixed and moving surfaces using the concave-convex rule.

- You should identify the techniques of roll, spin, and glide.

- You should describe and perform patient positioning and therapist hand placement for various joint mobilizations using good body mechanics.

- You should demonstrate loose- versus close-packed position of the shoulder.

- You should perform graded oscillations using good body mechanics.

Name_____ Date_____

Activities

1. Fill in the following chart using the concave-convex rule to joints where the fixed segment and the direction of movement are given.

Joint	Fixed	Action	Moving surface	Roll	Glide
Glenohumeral	glenoid	ABD	convex	superior	inferior
Glenohumeral	glenoid	ER			
Humeroulnar	humerus	EXT			
Radiocarpal	radius	FLE			
Second MCP	metacarpal	EXT			
Tibiofemoral	tibia	EXT			
Radiocarpal	radius	ADD			
Thumb IP	prox. phal.	FLE			

2. While wearing shorts and T-shirts, perform each of the glides listed in the chart on a partner. Be sure to use good body mechanics. Follow the instructions for each glide as described in the textbook.

3. For each of the following case studies, practice and demonstrate graded oscillations for the specific joint and direction(s). Select a partner to practice the following techniques on. For your first experience, use another person similar to you in body type and stature if possible. First, use a goniometer to measure each joint's beginning ROM. Then, practice joint mobilization on your partner using the scenarios described in the following case studies. Demonstrate to your instructor proper patient positioning, hand placements, body alignment, loose- versus close-packed positions, and graded oscillations.

Finally, how would you assess the effectiveness of your treatment?

Case A. Tom had arthroscopic knee surgery 48 h ago for a lateral release in his left knee. He now presents with decreased knee flexion.

1. Is his problem at the patellofemoral or at the knee joint?

2. Which gliding or rolling motion is probably giving him the most trouble?

3. What would be the purpose or goal of performing joint mobilizations on this patient?

4. How much motion would you expect him to gain?

Case B. Irene has just had a cast, which extended to her midforearm, removed following right thumb reconstructive surgery. Her radiocarpal joint is stiff.

1. What would be the purpose or goal of performing joint mobilizations on this patient?

2. How much motion would you expect her to gain?

Case C. Shawn has been immobilized in a sling due to a left elbow hyperextension injury sustained while wrestling. Now his shoulder has decreased abduction. Demonstrate longitudinal caudal (lateral [dis]traction) to his shoulder.

What would be the purpose or goal of performing traction on this patient?

Case D. Forty-year-old Susan strained her right rotator cuff in a water skiing accident two months ago. Thinking the pain would subside on its own, she simply rested her arm. Now she presents with limited abduction of the right shoulder to 55°. Demonstrate inferior glides to her glenohumeral joint while she is supine and abducted to 45°.

1. What would be the purpose or goal of performing joint mobilizations on this patient?

2. Will this position increase her ROM?

3. How will you know when you can increase her joint position to make the treatment progressive?

4. What new position will you choose?

LAB 6

Myofascial Release, Myofascial Trigger Points, and Muscle Energy

The purpose of this lab is to introduce you to, and provide practice sessions for learning, myofascial release, myofascial trigger point, and muscle energy techniques.

Review material from chapter 6 of the textbook before completing this lab.

OBJECTIVES

- You should understand indications and contra-indications and explain precautions for myofascial release, myofascial trigger point, and muscle energy techniques.

- You should know how to perform the basic techniques associated with myofascial release using good body mechanics.

- You should understand how to perform a trigger point examination.

- You should know how to perform the basic techniques associated with myofascial trigger points using good body mechanics.

- You should understand how to perform muscle energy techniques using good body mechanics.

Name_____   Date_____

Activities

1. Using a partner, practice performing the more common strokes and techniques associated with myofascial release—J strokes, oscillations, wringing, stripping, and leg pull. Practice and demonstrate myofascial release techniques using good body mechanics. Assume that your partner has muscle spasm preventing full knee extension following a quad strain. Palpate the structure, progressing from superficial to deep pressure. With either the finger pads, knuckles, thumb, or heel of the hand, apply a low-load force. The stabilizing hand should anchor the tissue proximal to the injured site and take up the slack. Draw a short J across the restricted area. Continue for 90 s. Next apply an oscillation to the area for 90 s. Try the wringing technique for 90 s. Going deeper, apply the stripping technique for 90 s. Finally, apply a longitudinal leg pull with your partner in supine. Traction is applied as the leg is moved slowly into abduction and rotation. Hold the position when tissue resistance is felt. As the tension releases, repeat the movement.

   A. Was one technique more effective than another?

   B. How can you tell?

   C. How can you determine if your treatment was effective?

   D. What tools would you need?

   E. What would you have to change to make the treatment more effective?

   F. Get feedback from your partner.

   G. Was there any discomfort as the treatment was being performed?

   H. How is the discomfort described?

   I. What can be done to alleviate the discomfort?

2. Using a partner, practice a trigger point examination. Because most of us carry some tension in our neck and shoulders, perform a compression test looking for taut muscle tissue over the levator scapulae and trapezius muscles. Locate the affected muscle's trigger point. Begin at the distal insertion, and palpate the fiber as you progress toward the proximal insertion. Your partner will let you know when you find an area of increased tenderness. You should feel the ball of hardness within the taut band.

3. Practice performing the three basic techniques associated with myofascial trigger points—ice stroking, ischemic compression, and stripping—using good body mechanics. Use your partner's neck and shoulders. Treat your partner's trigger point using the ice stroking technique. Bring the affected part through its full ROM. While gradually and passively stretching the muscle, slowly sweep ice two or three times over the length of the muscle and the area of referred pain. Take up the slack as the muscle relaxes. Repeat, starting from the new position. Next try the ischemic compression technique. Apply pressure to the trigger point until the tension subsides. Follow the compression by stretching the affected muscle. Finally try the stripping technique. Slowly perform a deep-stroke massage with your fingertips moving from the distal to proximal end of the muscle. Each stroke should get progressively deeper.

   A. Was one technique more effective than another?

   B. How can you tell?

   C. How can you determine if your treatment was effective?

   D. What tools would you need?

   E. What would you have to change to make the treatment more effective?

   F. Get feedback from your partner.

   G. Was there any discomfort as the treatment was being performed?

   H. How is the discomfort described?

   I. What can be done to alleviate the discomfort?

4. Using the examples in the textbook, practice and demonstrate muscle energy technique with a partner. Perform isotonic muscle energy for a basketball player who has undergone an ACL reconstruction, and isometric technique for a soccer player with groin pain from a contusion to the anterior ilium. The assessment of the problem has been done for you. Place the joint in the proper position. Have your partner actively contract the appropriate muscles. Apply the appropriate counterforce. Apply the appropriate stretch force.

A. How can you determine if your treatment was effective?

B. What tools would you need?

C. What would you have to change to make the treatment more effective?

D. Get feedback from your partner.

E. Was there any discomfort as the treatment was being performed?

F. How is the discomfort described?

G. What can be done to alleviate the discomfort?

LAB 7

Muscle-Strengthening Exercises

The purpose of this lab is to help you apply the wide variety of muscle-strengthening exercises used in a clinical setting.

Review material from chapter 7 of the textbook before completing this lab.

OBJECTIVES

- You should distinguish between open and closed kinetic chain muscle-strengthening exercises.

- You should apply the SNAP principle to muscle-strengthening exercises.

- You should differentiate between and perform AROM, AAROM, PROM, and RROM.

- You should plan body-weight strengthening exercises.

- You should develop a therapeutic exercise protocol using rubber bands and tubing.

- You should be proficient in the use of free weights, including cuff weights, barbells, and dumbbells.

- You should understand when and how isotonic machines are used in therapeutic exercise.

Name_____   Date_____

Activities

1. Select a partner. Using manual muscle resistance, perform exercises to improve muscular strength of the wrist in all ranges. Perform two sets of 10 reps.

    A. Which type of ROM should you perform first, before providing manual muscle resistance?

    B. Where should you provide resistance?

    C. Why do you need to remind your patient to breathe?

    D. What should you do if your patient begins to use his or her elbow to help the movement?

2. Use a partner to practice manual muscle resistance exercises for the ankle. Perform two sets of 10 reps in each direction.

    A. Where should you provide resistance?

    B. How can you prevent your partner from using his or her knee?

3. Make a list of body-weight strengthening exercises for the shoulder. Put your list in order so that the easiest one comes first and the hardest one last.

Assuming you were going to use these exercises with a patient, how would you describe the type of ROM that should be performed first to assure proper technique?

4. Make up a body-weight strengthening exercise progression for the knee.

5. Using the list from activities 3 and 4, describe how you could make body-weight strengthening exercises progressive.

6. What instruction would you give a patient as he/she begins any exercise program that utilizes rubber bands or tubing?

7. Design a protocol using rubber bands or tubing for an ice hockey player who is trying to improve strength in his injured adductors and hip flexors. Be sure to include the SNAP principle.

8. Design a protocol using rubber bands or tubing for an injured baseball or softball player to improve his or her throwing strength. Be sure to include the SNAP principle.

9. Assume that you have a variety of free-weight exercise equipment (cuff weights, barbells, and dumbbells) in your rehabilitation setting. Design one open kinetic chain resistive exercise progression to improve strength around the knee, and another for the elbow. Remember to take into account the relationship between the pull of gravity on the weight and the position of the knee and the elbow as you work through your rehabilitation progression. Following the SNAP principle, be sure to include sets and reps.

A. At what point in your progression would you change from free-weight exercises to isotonic exercises?

B. What effect will performing an isometric contraction in some part of the ROM have on the muscle's strength?

C. As a rehabilitation specialist, what is the best way for you to ensure that the athlete is able to perform the exercise correctly?

LAB 8

Isokinetics—Using a Dynamometer

The purpose of this lab is to familiarize you with how isokinetic dynamometers work and how to integrate isokinetic exercise into therapeutic exercise.

Review material from chapter 7 of the textbook before completing this lab.

OBJECTIVES

- You should properly position the patient on an isokinetic dynamometer.

- You should set the dynamometer for testing, passive motion, submaximal and maximal exercise bouts.

Name_____   Date_____

Activities

1. Learn how to use an isokinetic dynamometer. Select a partner. Set up the dynamometer to test the knee. Set the dynamometer for concentric ROM to orient your partner to the specific exercise protocol, and perform three practice trials. Test the joint's strength using a slow and a fast speed. Forty-eight hours later, have your partner return for an exercise session. Again, set the dynamometer for concentric ROM to orient your partner to the specific exercise protocol. Using the same joint and setup, complete a submaximal and a maximal exercise bout. Print out your results.

2. Practice your dynamometer setups by completing each of the following scenarios. Where applicable include passive motion, testing, and submaximal and maximal exercise bouts.

   Case A. An 18-year-old college basketball player wants to get his ankles taped. He explains that he had numerous sprains in high school and would like support for his "weak" ankles. You decide that a two-speed isokinetic program would increase his strength.

   • Using a dynamometer, test the athlete's ankle strength.

   • Design an exercise protocol to include both concentric and eccentric strength training. Test your design on a partner. Print out your results.

   Case B. Sue is a 21-year-old junior soccer player. She sustained a grade II hip flexor strain of her right (dominant) leg during the middle of her season. Rehabilitation consisted of ice, electric stimulation, and Theraband strengthening exercises. Her strength has returned, but her ability to produce a strong shot on goal remains weak. She is anxious to regain her power and agrees to an off-season rehabilitation program.

   Using the dynamometer, design an exercise protocol to increase hip flexor power. Be sure to include both concentric and eccentric exercise bouts. Test your design on a partner. Print out your results.

   Case C. The baseball season is fast approaching. The pitching coach has come to you and asked if an isokinetic strengthening program would help solve some of last year's baseball pitchers' sore shoulders.

   Realizing that deceleration is most likely the cause of the majority of the problem, you decide to design an exercise protocol on a dynamometer to work the rotator cuff. Test your design on a partner. Print out your results.

   Case D. John is a first-year student playing on the varsity tennis team. He has developed tennis elbow from all the backhand drills he has been doing in practice. The coach has evaluated and made adjustments to John's technique.

   Design an isokinetic exercise protocol to improve John's strength. Test your design on a partner. Print out your results.

3. Answer the following questions:

   A. What are the advantages of isokinetic testing and exercise?

   B. How can an isokinetic dynamometer be used for tendinitis?

LAB 9

Proprioceptive Neuromuscular Facilitation

The purpose of this lab is to provide you with controlled, practical applications for PNF technique. Review material from chapter 7 of the textbook before completing this lab.

OBJECTIVES

- You should perform proper hand placement when applying PNF patterns.

- You should utilize proper verbal cues when applying PNF patterns.

- You should give brief and concise instruction when initiating PNF patterns with a patient.

- You should allow for smooth patient movement when performing PNF patterns.

- You should demonstrate good body mechanics when applying PNF patterns.

- You should understand and demonstrate PNF patterns used to develop strength, endurance, and coordination.

- You should understand and demonstrate PNF patterns used to increase ROM, relaxation, and inhibition.

- You should understand and demonstrate diagonal patterns to the shoulder, hip, upper trunk, and lower trunk.

Name_____ Date_____

Activities

1. The men's basketball team at your university always seem to have poor hamstring flexibility. You decide to test the three PNF techniques that are used to increase ROM, relaxation, and inhibition to find out which technique you should recommend to improve that component of fitness. Those techniques are contract-relax, hold-relax, and slow reversal-hold-relax. Select a partner. Practice all three techniques to determine which one you should recommend. Remember to start with rhythmic initiation.

2. Compare the three techniques.

   A. Was one easier to do than another?

   B. Which one?

   C. Why?

   D. For which technique did your partner show the most gains?

   E. Therefore, which technique would you recommend the basketball team use to increase their flexibility?

3. You had so much success with the basketball team in the earlier scenario that you decide to use PNF with the women's swim team to help develop their rotator cuffs for strength, endurance, and coordination. The four PNF techniques used to develop those fitness components are repeated contraction, slow reversal, slow reversal-hold, and rhythmic stabilization. Select a partner. Practice all four techniques to determine which one you should recommend. Remember to start with rhythmic initiation.

4. Compare the four techniques.

   A. Was one easier to do than another?

   B. Which one?

C. Why?

D. For which technique did your partner show the most gains?

E. Therefore, which technique would you recommend the swim team use to increase their strength?

5. Practice each of the four diagonal patterns on both sides of the body using rhythmic initiation. The four patterns are shoulder, hip, upper trunk, and lower trunk. Then perform the slow-reversal PNF technique in each of those patterns.

6. Answer the following questions:

A. Did you find any differences on one side of the body compared to the other?

B. What were they?

C. What made practicing these patterns difficult for you?

D. What made practicing these patterns difficult for your partner?

E. What were your limitations in performing these patterns?

7. Give two examples of injuries for which you would recommend diagonal patterns for each of the four body areas.

A. Hip

B. Shoulder

C. Upper trunk

D. Lower trunk

LAB 10

Proprioception and Neuromuscular Control

The purpose of this lab is to provide you with opportunities to practice the assessment of neuromuscular control and reposition sense.

Review material from chapter 8 of the textbook before completing this lab.

OBJECTIVES

- You should be able to assess static and dynamic balance.

- You should assess proprioception (reposition sense) using several different methods.

- You should assess two-point discrimination.

Name_____ Date_____

Activities

1. **Neuromuscular Control.** Work with a partner. For all the following tests, your partner will perform 30-s trials using the leg that he/she would **not** choose when kicking a ball. Count each error during the 30-s test for a total Error Score (ES). Record errors as listed in the scoring chart below. Each error is scored as 1.

   This lab is as much for the scorer as for the subject. Practice being consistent in determining errors. You should stand directly in front of or behind your partner when scoring.

   For tests A through C, keep arms crossed over chest and keep contralateral leg in tight to test leg (i.e., thighs adducted).

   A. Modified Romberg (for knee/hip)   Error Score _____

   EYES CLOSED. Single-limb balance, hip and knee slightly flexed, non-weight-bearing leg bent to approximately 45° to 50°, arms crossed. Hold for 30 s.

   B. Modified Romberg (for ankle)   Error Score _____

   EYES CLOSED. Single-limb balance, hip and knee fully extended (force corrections at ankle), non-weight-bearing leg bent to approximately 45° to 50°, arms held in tight or crossed. Hold for 30 s.

   C. Sharpened Romberg   Error Score _____

   EYES CLOSED. Stand with one foot in front of the other (in a heel-to-toe position). Place your nonpreferred (i.e., nonkicking) leg in the rear. Keep arms in tight and knees and hips fully extended. Hold for 30 s.

   D. Functional hop test   Error Score _____

Equipment needed: *tape measure, tape, felt-tip marker*

   Set up area according to the following chart. Have your partner hop to each of the numbers starting on number 1. Upon landing, he/she should immediately bring arms to side and fully extend knee and hip. Maintain balance for 5 s before hopping to the next number. Use the scoring system shown in the following box.

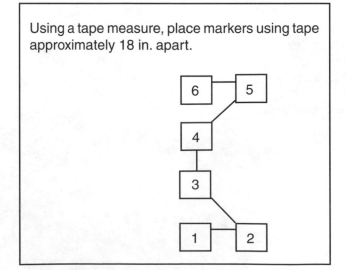

Using a tape measure, place markers using tape approximately 18 in. apart.

Scoring—Error Score (ES)

30-s trial

Count one error each time one of the following occurs:

- moves test foot or doesn't "stick" the landing
- doesn't hold for full 5 s on each number
- moves arm for balance
- contralateral leg moves away from test leg
- touches down contralateral leg
- body sways > 4 in. in any direction

2. **Proprioception (Reposition Sense).** Five different methods of assessing reposition sense are given here. Instructors are encouraged to have students use any or all of the methods described. Students should perform three trials of each test.

  A. Active shoulder rotation using goniometer

Equipment needed: *goniometer, treatment table*

Using a goniometer attached to a table, measure shoulder rotation proprioception. Position your partner so that the shoulder joint is in line with the axis of the goniometer. Use 90° to the table as neutral. Your partner's eyes should be closed during the test trials. Have your partner move his/her arm into internal rotation and hold for 5 s, concentrating on the position. Have him/her move back to start and then try to replicate the same position. You will note the degrees of error in the second trial by comparing with the first trial (i.e., if on the first trial internal rotation was 30° and on the second trial it was 27°, the "error" is 3°).

Starting ROM_____

  1st trial _____   _____ degrees of error (ROM ± 1st trial)

  2nd trial _____   _____ degrees of error (ROM ± 2nd trial)

  3rd trial _____   _____ degrees of error (ROM ± 3rd trial)

                              _____ average of degrees of error

  B. Active knee extension using inclinometer

Equipment needed: *table, bubble inclinometer or angle finder (can be purchased from hardware store for $4.00–$8.00)*

Using a bubble inclinometer (or angle finder), measure knee extension proprioception. Your partner should be seated on a treatment table with knee flexed to 90°. Your partner will actively perform (eyes closed) knee extension to about 45° with the inclinometer held on the anterior lower leg. He or she should hold this position for 5 s, then move back to flexion and immediately attempt to replicate the position. You will note the error in the second trial by comparing with the first trial.

Starting ROM_____

  1st trial _____   _____ degrees of error (ROM ± 1st trial)

  2nd trial _____   _____ degrees of error (ROM ± 2nd trial)

  3rd trial _____   _____ degrees of error (ROM ± 3rd trial)

                              _____ average of degrees of error

C. Weight-bearing ankle inversion using inclinometer

Equipment needed: *inclinometer and wobble or tilt board*

Have your partner stand on the wobble or tilt board with the inclinometer attached to the board. Your partner will invert his/her foot to a position of choice. He/she will hold this position for 5 s, then move back to neutral and immediately attempt to replicate the original inversion position. You will note the error in degrees.

Starting ROM_____

1st trial _____	_____ degrees of error (ROM ± 1st trial)
2nd trial _____	_____ degrees of error (ROM ± 2nd trial)
3rd trial _____	_____ degrees of error (ROM ± 3rd trial)
	_____ average of degrees of error

D. Non-weight-bearing proprioception using isokinetic dynamometer

Equipment needed: *isokinetic dynamometer*

Using an isokinetic device, set up the device according to manufacturer's specifications for the particular joint and motion you wish to assess. You must be in a setting that will allow you to read the degrees of joint motion as it takes place. If you cannot see the ROM, follow the directions at the end of this section. Follow the same procedure as described for the three previous methods.

If you cannot see degrees of motion: During setup of the device, most isokinetic dynamometers go through a phase in which you set the "zero" range of motion. At this point you will be able to see degrees of motion. You may perform your proprioception assessment here. Movement of the device causes the internal goniometer to register the ROM in degrees.

Starting ROM_____

1st trial _____	_____ degrees of error (ROM ± 1st trial)
2nd trial _____	_____ degrees of error (ROM ± 2nd trial)
3rd trial _____	_____ degrees of error (ROM ± 3rd trial)
	_____ average of degrees of error

E. Weight-bearing knee flexion using digital photography

Equipment needed: *reflective balls, circular stickers, or felt-tip marker; digital camera; computer and printer; small clear goniometer or protractor*

Place markers (reflective balls, circular stickers) over the lateral malleolus, lateral knee joint just above the fibular head, and the greater trochanter. You must have an unobstructed side view of your partner. Have your partner perform knee/hip flexion to a midrange of motion and hold for 5 s. Take a picture. Have your partner move to standing position and repeat the test; take a picture when your partner says he/she believes him-/herself to be back in the test position. Print out the pictures and measure the knee ROM using a goniometer or protractor, aligning the axis with the knee marker and the arms of the goniometer with the malleolus and greater trochanter markers.

Starting ROM_____

1st trial _____	_____ degrees of error (ROM ± 1st trial)
2nd trial _____	_____ degrees of error (ROM ± 2nd trial)
3rd trial _____	_____ degrees of error (ROM ± 3rd trial)
	_____ average of degrees of error

1. How is joint position related to postural sway (balance)? In other words, why do we assess postural sway when we are interested in proprioception?

2. Would you expect to see a relationship between reposition sense of the ankle and postural sway?

3. If you were conducting a study to determine the effect of a neoprene sleeve on ankle joint proprioception and were using balance as a measure, how would you position the subjects and what directions would you give them to better ensure you were measuring "ankle" input?

3. Cutaneous Two-Point Discrimination

Equipment needed: *two-point discriminator or paperclips straightened and bent to increasing widths of 0.5 to 5 cm (0.2–2 in.)*

Measure two-point discrimination at various sites: anterior forearm, great toe, index finger, and low back. With your partner's eyes closed, assess two-point discrimination by randomly selecting discriminator widths (0.5–5 cm). When the two points do not make contact simultaneously, the number of points is obvious, so be sure to make contact with both points simultaneously. Your partner will state whether he/she feels one point or two. Compare the difference between forearm, great toe (pad), finger (pad), and low back.

Forearm

Great toe (pad)

Finger (pad)

Low back

A. Which area had the most discriminating sense?

B. Is this as you expected?

LAB 11

Plyometrics

The purpose of this lab is to prepare you to assess the effectiveness of plyometric exercise and to formulate plyometric progressions based on that assessment.

Review material from chapter 9 of the textbook before completing this lab.

OBJECTIVES

- You should understand the effects of speed during the prestretch and amortization phases of plyometrics.

- You should use appropriate body position to perform plyometrics.

- You should formulate plyometric progressions for the lower and upper extremity and the trunk.

Name_____ Date_____

Activities

1. Get into pairs. Using a vertical jump assessment device, perform a series of jumps to compare the effects of a quick versus a slow prestretch and amortization period. Perform each of the following jumps once, measure each jump, and record the results. Begin each jump from a standing position.

   Jump 1: Quickly bend your knees to approximately 60° and jump.

   Jump 2: Slowly bend your knees to approximately 60°, hold for 3 s, and jump.

   Jump 3: Quickly bend your knees to approximately 120° and jump.

   Jump 4: Slowly bend your knees to approximately 120°, hold for 3 s, and jump.

   A. Results: How high did you jump?

   Jump 1:

   Jump 2:

   Jump 3:

   Jump 4:

   B. Which jump produced the greatest height?

   C. Why?

2. Now perform a series of jumps to determine the most advantageous body position and arm movement during the jump, as well as proper foot placement on landing for optimal force production. Repeat each jump from the preceding example, adding the following conditions. Perform five jumps using each condition. Record your average jump height in the table below.

   Condition 1: Use no arms; land on the balls of your feet.

   Condition 2: Use your arms; land on the balls of your feet.

   Condition 3: Use your arms; land on your midfoot.

   A. Results: How high did you jump?

	Condition 1	Condition 2	Condition 3
Jump 1			
Jump 2			
Jump 3			
Jump 4			

    B. Which jump produced the greatest height?

    C. Why?

3. For each of the following case studies, design a progression for the lower extremity (using jumps-in-place, standing jumps, multiple jumps and hops, bounding, box drills, and depth jumps), or a progression for the upper extremity and trunk (using weighted balls), to fit each individual's needs. Be sure to include how each athlete should progress through his or her program.

    Case A. Jennifer is a 20-year-old rugby player participating in a preseason conditioning program. Design a plyometric program for her to improve her leg power.

Case B. Jeff is a 16-year-old volleyball player who has been rehabilitating a second-degree right ankle sprain. List the test(s) you would perform to see if he is able to withstand the stresses of a plyometric program. Design a program based on your results.

Case C. Heather is an 18-year-old freestyle swimmer. She competes in the short distances, including relays. She is beginning to complain of shoulder muscle soreness after every practice. She admits that she has been swimming more laps than she had in high school. In addition to ice and shoulder stretching exercises, you decide that a plyometric program will provide her with the necessary shoulder strength to compete at the collegiate level. What test(s) will you complete to determine her readiness for plyometrics? Design a program based on your results.

Case D. Eli is a 44-year-old who has been referred to your rehabilitation clinic for abdominal-strengthening exercises. He was diagnosed with a low back strain caused by overuse while performing his job at UPS. He has progressed through the first three phases of a pelvic stabilization program that includes abdominal curls and back extension exercises. To add variety to his program, you decide to include plyometric exercises. Design a program to fit his trunk strength.

Functional Progressions

The purpose of this lab is to present you with the concept of applying functional progressions in rehabilitation programs.

Review material from chapter 10 of the textbook before completing this lab.

OBJECTIVES

- You should understand the difference between basic and advanced functional exercise progressions.

- You should describe the components of advanced functional progressions—force/intensity, speed, distance, complexity, and support.

- You should be able to explain to the patient the precautions associated with functional progressions.

Name_____ Date_____

Activities

1. For each case study described, create a functional exercise protocol. Use as much variety as possible in your programs by including many different types of exercises (open and closed kinetic chains) and rehabilitation tools (Theraband, free weights, PNF, aquatics, etc.). Begin by listing all the potential functional exercises you would like to see included in each rehabilitation protocol. Then go back through your list and indicate how you will include the components of an advanced functional progression (force/intensity, speed, distance, complexity, and support).

   Case A. Paulo is a high school ice hockey goalie. As he was attempting to make a save, a forward from the opposing team collided with him. He suffered a grade II sprain to his left anterior talofibular and calcaneofibular ligaments, with accompanying strains to the everter muscles. Twenty-four hours later he is 50% weight bearing and has substantial swelling and ecchymosis.

   Describe your functional exercise protocol. In other words, what exercises will you begin with? It has been two weeks and Paulo is able to bear full weight without pain. How will you progress?

Case B. Angela is a college senior diagnosed with a grade III acromioclavicular right shoulder separation and associated deltoid and trapezius muscle strain. Her mechanism of injury was a fall on the tip of her right shoulder from an inadvertent collision during an early-season lacrosse game. She is right-handed. Having been immobilized for two weeks, she is now ready for rehabilitation.

Describe your functional exercise protocol. In other words, what exercises will you begin with? Three weeks later, Angela's strength and ROM are ready for more advanced rehabilitation. How will you progress?

2. Answer the following questions.

   A. How soon can you begin functional exercise?

   B. What functional tests will Paulo and Angela have to perform to allow them to return to full practice and competition?

LAB 13

Posture Analysis

The purpose of this lab is to prepare you to perform posture screening.

Review material from chapter 11 of the textbook before completing this lab.

OBJECTIVES

- You should recognize postural abnormalities and identify possible chronic pathologies related to those abnormalities.

Name_____   Date_____

Activities

Working in groups of four, perform postural assessment of each group member using the forms included here. Identify postural abnormalities and develop exercise treatment protocols for each individual based on your findings. For this lab, students should wear shorts; females should wear a bathing-suit top or tank top.

Equipment needed: *plumb line or wall grid, postural assessment sheet, digital camera if available*

The student being observed should stand behind a plumb line or in front of a wall grid. Observers should position themselves in line with the individual and approximately 3 m to 4.5 m (10–15 ft) away. You will observe each student from the front, back, and side. For each view, begin with the feet and work your way up. Note any malalignments on the screening form. At the end of the form, write your assessment and any plans for corrective exercise treatment or postural training. If a digital camera is available, take a photo from each direction, print the photos, and share your findings with the individual. Repeat for each member of the group. Use the following form to aid in documenting your findings.

Postural Screening

Front View	**Front View**

Front View

Front View

Overall alignment
Vertical alignment
Plumb line should be equidistant between feet.

- [ ] pubic symphysis
- [ ] umbilicus
- [ ] xiphoid
- [ ] sternal notch
- [ ] tip of nose

Horizontal alignment

- [ ] medial malleoli height
- [ ] patella height
- [ ] ASIS height (if not =, measure real leg length)
- [ ] acromion height

Foot/ankle
L R B   [ ] pes planus   [ ] pes cavus
L R B   [ ] forefoot valgus [ ] varus
L R B   [ ] hallux valgus   [ ] hammer-/claw toes

Fick angle _____

Knees
L R B   [ ] genu valgus   [ ] genu varus

Tibial rotation
L R B   [ ] internal   [ ] external

Hips
Femoral rotation
L R B   [ ] anteversion   [ ] retroversion

Shoulders
Humeral rotation
L R B   [ ] internal   [ ] external

Trunk rotation_____   Head rotation_____   Lat. flex._____

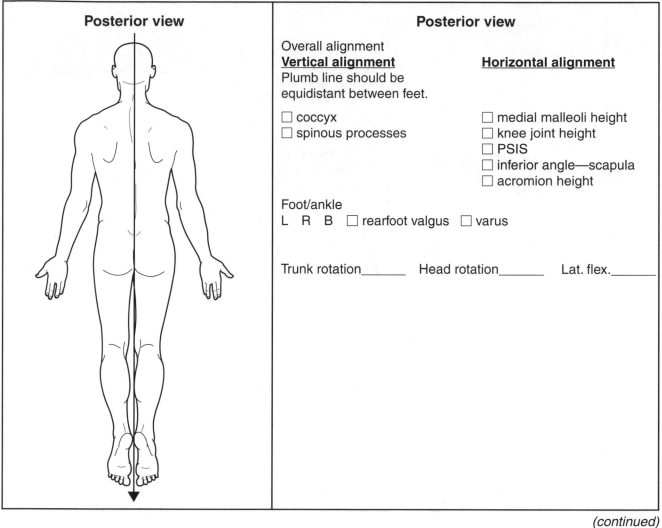

Posterior view

Posterior view

Overall alignment

| **Vertical alignment** | **Horizontal alignment** |

Plumb line should be equidistant between feet.

☐ coccyx
☐ spinous processes

☐ medial malleoli height
☐ knee joint height
☐ PSIS
☐ inferior angle—scapula
☐ acromion height

Foot/ankle
L   R   B   ☐ rearfoot valgus   ☐ varus

Trunk rotation_____   Head rotation_____   Lat. flex._____

(continued)

Side view	Side view

Overall alignment

Vertical alignment	**Horizontal alignment**
Plumb line should be just anterior to lateral malleolus.	

☐ mid-knee joint   ☐ pelvic tilt
☐ greater trochanter   ☐ lordosis
☐ acromion process   ☐ kyphosis
☐ inferior tip of ear   ☐ forward-head posture
                            ☐ flat back
                            ☐ military posture

Foot/ankle
L   R   B   ☐ dorsi-   ☐ plantar

Knees
L   R   B   ☐ genu recurvatum

Hips
L   R   B   ☐ flexed

Shoulders
L   R   B   ☐ flexion   ☐ extension

Elbows
L   R   B   ☐ carrying angle

Assessment:

Plan:

Human body illustrations reprinted, by permission, from P.A. Houglum, 2001, *Therapeutic Exercise for Athletic Injuries* (Champaign, IL: Human Kinetics), 169.

LAB 14

Gait Analysis and Ambulation Aids

The purpose of this lab is to prepare you to perform gait analysis with and without ambulation aids. Review material from chapter 12 of the textbook before completing this lab.

OBJECTIVES

- You should identify normal gait patterns.

- You should recognize gait disturbances and identify possible chronic pathologies related to those abnormalities.

- You should inspect and adjust axillary and forearm crutches, and canes, for proper patient fit.

- You should differentiate between three-point gait, four-point gait, and single-support patterns.

- You should know how to use assistive devices on stairs and ramps and in transfers.

Name_____ Date_____

Activities

1. Working in the same groups of four as for the posture lab, review your previously acquired postural findings. Make a list of gait disturbances that you may expect to observe on the basis of your findings from the postural assessment.

2. Perform gait analysis of each group member using the following form. Identify gait disturbances and develop a treatment plan for each individual based on your findings.

Student #1 _____

Front/Back View

Heel contact	☐ yes	☐ no	tibial external rotation	☐ yes	☐ no	foot supination
Midstance	☐ yes	☐ no	tibial internal rotation	☐ yes	☐ no	foot pronation
Heel-off	☐ yes	☐ no	tibial internal rotation	☐ yes	☐ no	foot pronation
Toe-off	☐ yes	☐ no	tibial external rotation	☐ yes	☐ no	foot supination

Side View

Heel contact	☐ yes	☐ no	tibial external rotation	☐ yes	☐ no	foot supination
Midstance	☐ yes	☐ no	tibial internal rotation	☐ yes	☐ no	foot pronation
Heel-off	☐ yes	☐ no	tibial internal rotation	☐ yes	☐ no	foot pronation
Toe-off	☐ yes	☐ no	tibial external rotation	☐ yes	☐ no	foot supination

Student #2 _____

Front/Back View

Heel contact	☐ yes	☐ no	tibial external rotation	☐ yes	☐ no	foot supination
Midstance	☐ yes	☐ no	tibial internal rotation	☐ yes	☐ no	foot pronation
Heel-off	☐ yes	☐ no	tibial internal rotation	☐ yes	☐ no	foot pronation
Toe-off	☐ yes	☐ no	tibial external rotation	☐ yes	☐ no	foot supination

Side View

Heel contact	☐ yes	☐ no	tibial external rotation	☐ yes	☐ no	foot supination
Midstance	☐ yes	☐ no	tibial internal rotation	☐ yes	☐ no	foot pronation
Heel-off	☐ yes	☐ no	tibial internal rotation	☐ yes	☐ no	foot pronation
Toe-off	☐ yes	☐ no	tibial external rotation	☐ yes	☐ no	foot supination

Student #3 _____

Front/Back View

Heel contact	☐ yes	☐ no	tibial external rotation	☐ yes	☐ no	foot supination
Midstance	☐ yes	☐ no	tibial internal rotation	☐ yes	☐ no	foot pronation
Heel-off	☐ yes	☐ no	tibial internal rotation	☐ yes	☐ no	foot pronation
Toe-off	☐ yes	☐ no	tibial external rotation	☐ yes	☐ no	foot supination

Side View

Heel contact	☐ yes	☐ no	tibial external rotation	☐ yes	☐ no	foot supination
Midstance	☐ yes	☐ no	tibial internal rotation	☐ yes	☐ no	foot pronation
Heel-off	☐ yes	☐ no	tibial internal rotation	☐ yes	☐ no	foot pronation
Toe-off	☐ yes	☐ no	tibial external rotation	☐ yes	☐ no	foot supination

---

3. Select a partner. Inspect and adjust axillary and forearm crutches, as well as a cane, to fit your partner. Instruct him or her in the proper use of crutches and canes for three-point gait, four-point gait, and single-support gait patterns. Practice using the assistive devices on stairs and ramps and in transfer. When you feel confident, have your partner use the following checklist to test your proficiency.

Inspect and adjust axillary crutches

☐ checks crutch screws for tightness

☐ checks crutch tips for wear

☐ checks crutch pads for wear

☐ places tip 15 cm (6 in.) from outer margin of shoe

☐ places tip 15 cm in front of shoe

☐ measures axillary brace so that it is 2.5 cm (1 in.) below anterior fold of axilla

☐ measures hand brace so that elbow is at 30°

Inspect and adjust forearm crutches

☐ checks crutch screws for tightness

☐ checks crutch tips for wear

☐ checks crutch pads for wear

☐ places tip 15 cm (6 in.) from outer margin of shoe

☐ places tip 15 cm in front of shoe

☐ measures handgrip to be at the level of the greater trochanter

☐ measures forearm cuff to be just distal to the elbow

☐ measures hand brace so that elbow is at 30°

Walking with crutches—tripod/swing-through method (non-weight bearing)

☐ instructs athlete to stand on one foot with the affected foot completely elevated

☐ instructs athlete to place crutch tips 30 cm to 38 cm (12–15 in.) ahead of feet

☐ instructs athlete to keep injured leg in line with the crutches

☐ reminds athlete to not put weight on axilla pad

☐ instructs athlete to straighten the elbows

☐ instructs athlete to step through crutches with noninjured leg

☐ instructs athlete to recover crutches and place tips forward for next step

☐ gives safety instructions for throw rugs, slippery surfaces, obstacles

Walking with crutches—partial-weight-bearing method

☐ instructs athlete to take as much weight as is pain free on injured leg

☐ instructs athlete to take the rest of body weight on hands

☐ reminds athlete to not put weight on axilla pad

☐ instructs athlete to place crutch tips 30 cm to 38 cm (12–15 in.) ahead of feet

☐ instructs athlete to lean forward, straighten the elbows, and step through

☐ instructs athlete to keep injured leg in line with the crutches

☐ instructs athlete to recover crutches and place tips forward for next step

☐ gives safety instructions for throw rugs, slippery surfaces, obstacles

Walking with crutch—four-point gait method

☐ instructs athlete to stand on both feet

☐ instructs athlete to move one crutch forward (L)

☐ instructs athlete to step forward with opposite foot (R)

☐ instructs athlete to move crutch on opposite side just ahead of foot (R)

☐ instructs athlete to step forward with other foot (L)

☐ gives safety instructions for throw rugs, slippery surfaces, obstacles

Inspect and fit canes

☐ checks cane tips for wear

☐ checks cane grip for wear

☐ measures cane height with arm relaxed and resting at the side

☐ measures cane height with cane next to the side, handle at waist level

Single-support (crutch or cane) instruction

☐ places support on correct side in relation to injury limb

☐ instructs the athlete to move the crutch/cane and the injured limb together

☐ reminds the athlete to apply weight to the crutch/cane as the uninvolved leg moves forward

☐ gives safety instructions for throw rugs, slippery surfaces, obstacles

Climbing stairs

☐ instructs athlete to use the handrail

☐ instructs athlete to remain in an upright position

☐ instructs athlete in rule—"up with the good, down with the bad" (must interpret rule) —or—

☐ instructs athlete that the assistive device always goes with the involved leg

Using a ramp

☐ instructs athlete to remain in an upright position

☐ instructs athlete that the assistive device always goes with the involved leg

☐ instructs athlete to take short steps

Transferring from a chair (two crutches, one crutch or cane)

☐ instructs athlete to hold assistive device with one hand on the handgrips

☐ instructs athlete to place the crutches vertically near but in front and to the side of the chair

☐ instructs athlete to place the other hand on the chair's arm or seat

☐ instructs athlete to stand up and reposition assistive device before proceeding

LAB 15

Aquatic Therapy

The purpose of this lab is to present you with the concepts of aquatic therapy and to provide controlled practice in aquatic therapy situations. Review material from chapter 13 of the textbook before completing this lab.

OBJECTIVES

- You should differentiate between form drag and wave drag.

- You should explain and perform aquatic exercises for the trunk, neck, lower extremity, and upper extremity in both deep and shallow water.

Name_____ Date_____

Activities

1. Experience form drag. Standing in shallow water, move your hand through the water, changing the position of the palm. First, move the hand through the water with the palm parallel to the water's surface. Keep the fingers together. Now change the position of the hand so that it is perpendicular to the water's surface. Move the hand, first keeping the fingers opened, then keeping them closed. If one is available, hold onto a hand paddle, and move the hand perpendicular to the water's surface. Now move your whole arm across the water's surface.

   Why is each of these exercises more progressive in nature?

2. Experience wave drag. While walking across the shallow end of the pool, repeat all of the preceding exercises. Increase your pace to a run while moving the hand.

   Why do these exercises become increasingly difficult?

3. For each of the following case studies, create and demonstrate a four-phase aquatic therapy program. In all cases the physician has cleared the patient for participation in an aquatic therapy program. None of the patients are afraid of the water, and all can swim. Where appropriate, list which assistive and/or resistive devices you would need. You are not limited to the exercises listed in the text, but use them where applicable.

   Case A. A 39-year-old female has chronic low back pain. She also has weak abdominal muscles.

Case B. A 25-year-old male is recovering from whiplash. The injury is limited to the neck extensors and rotators.

Case C. A 20-year-old football player has a second-degree left syndesmosis sprain. Swelling is minimal, yet he is still only partially weight bearing.

Case D. A 19-year-old wrestler had surgery 10 days ago to repair a Bankart lesion in his right shoulder.

LAB 16

Swiss Balls and Foam Rollers

The purpose of this lab is to prepare you to use Swiss balls and foam rollers in therapeutic exercise sessions.

Review material from chapter 14 of the textbook before completing this lab.

OBJECTIVE

- You should understand the precautions, indications, and contraindications for using Swiss balls and foam rollers.

Name_____ Date_____

Activities

1. Select a partner for each of the following trunk and lower- and upper-extremity exercises. Practice giving explicit directions, as well as spotting when necessary. Follow the directions for each exercise as described in the chapter.

   A. Practice each of the following exercises for the trunk using a Swiss ball:
   - Bounce and kick
   - Side foot reach
   - Lateral glide
   - Pelvic curls
   - Trunk rotation in sitting
   - Trunk rotation in supine
   - Stretch in kneeling
   - Lateral stretch
   - Thoracic stretch
   - Back extension in prone
   - Supine leg lift
   - Hip rotation
   - Bridging (both positions)
   - Prone leg lift
   - Swimming
   - Seated abdominal strengthening
   - Ball lift
   - Side sit-ups
   - Prone walk-out

   B. Practice each of the following exercises for the lower extremity using a Swiss ball:
   - Side leg lift
   - Half squat
   - Reverse squats
   - Hamstring curl
   - Side-lying ball lift
   - Ankle motion exercise

   C. Practice each of the following exercises for the upper extremity using a Swiss ball:
   - Prone flys
   - Triceps extension
   - Push-ups
   - Scapular retraction

D. Practice each of the following exercises for the trunk using foam rollers:
- Quadratus massage
- Thoracic massage
- Low back mobilization
- Cat stretch
- Quadruped balance
- Supine lower abdominal exercise
- Supine oblique exercise
- Abdominal crunch
- Rotational crunch
- Bridging
- Quadratus lumborum strengthening

E. Practice each of the following exercises for the lower extremity using foam rollers:
- Iliotibial band massage
- Quadriceps massage
- Standing balance
- Anterior tibialis stretch
- Gastrocnemius stretch
- Soleus stretch
- Piriformis stretch
- Squats

F. Practice each of the following exercises for the upper extremity using foam rollers:
- Arm stretches
- Push-ups
- Resistive band exercises in standing
- Resistive band exercises in supine
- Ball toss in supine
- Triceps press

2. Apply exercises outlined in the chapter to the following case studies, listing possible protocols a rehabilitation specialist might employ to treat injuries of the trunk and lower and upper extremities using Swiss balls and foam rollers.

Case A. Ming is a 15-year-old female gymnast diagnosed with a low back strain. Her physician would like you, her therapist, to set up a lumbar stabilization exercise program. You decide to include a Swiss ball and a foam roller.

Which exercises would you include in this protocol, and in what order?

Case B. Following a routine appendectomy, 19-year-old Bill has been cleared to begin an abdominal strengthening exercise program. While Bill's football season is over for this year, he is eager to participate in an off-season weight training program.

Using a Swiss ball and foam roller, list the exercises you would prescribe for him to get him ready to lift weights.

Case C. Jay separated his right AC joint during his first week of wrestling practice. His ROM and strength are such that you feel he is ready to begin scapulothoracic stabilization exercises.

Design an exercise protocol for this injury using a Swiss ball and foam roller.

Case D. You would like to add variety to Jorge's left ankle sprain exercise protocol.

Which Swiss-ball and foam-roller exercises can you add to his rehabilitation program?

LAB 17

Tendinitis

The purpose of this lab is to familiarize you with the special requirements of tendinitis rehabilitation.

Review material from chapter 15 of the textbook before completing this lab.

OBJECTIVE

- You should understand the special requirements of rehabilitation as it pertains to tendinitis.

Name_____   Date_____

Activities

Use the case studies described in chapter 15 to apply a functional rehabilitation protocol for injuries to the upper and lower extremities. The following is the challenge case study presented in chapter 15 of the textbook.

Case Study. Joe, a 19-year-old right-handed tennis player, presents with complaints of right elbow pain. The pain is located over the outside of the elbow and sometimes radiates down the forearm. It began about four months ago, about three weeks after Joe bought a new tennis racket and started playing in two leagues. He stopped playing for a month until he was pain free, but when he went back to playing, the pain returned. He plays or practices tennis daily. He has noticed that the elbow especially bothers him on his tennis backhand, when he attempts to lift heavy objects, and when he shakes hands with someone.

The right elbow and forearm have full ROM in all planes. The neck and shoulder also have normal motion. There is pain to resisted wrist extension. Joe's grip strength is weaker on the right than on the left by 6.8 kg (15 lb). Palpation of the lateral epicondyle reveals swelling over the epicondyle and tenderness to even light palpation. There is some tenderness to palpation extending into the proximal wrist extensor muscle bellies in the forearm.

1. What will be included in your first treatment session?

2. What will be your instructions to Joe concerning what he should and should not be doing at home?

3. How will you advance him in his program?

4. What exercises will you include?

LAB 18

Trunk Rehabilitation Protocol

The purpose of this lab is to give you practice utilizing various trunk therapeutic exercises and to present case studies specific to trunk rehabilitation. Review material from chapter 16 of the textbook before completing this lab.

OBJECTIVES

- You should understand how to apply trigger point and ice-and-stretch therapy to the cervical, thoracic, and lumbar spine.

- You should use flexibility exercises to relieve muscle pain in the cervical and thoracic spine.

- You should apply low back stabilization exercises.

- You should apply cervical, upper back, lower back, abdominal, and pelvis strengthening exercises.

- You should apply agility and coordination exercises.

- You should apply muscle energy techniques to lesions of the sacroiliac joint.

- You should understand how thoracic outlet syndrome can be treated with therapeutic exercises of the trunk.

Name_____   Date_____

Activities

1. For each of the following, select a partner. Follow the directions as given in chapter 16 of the textbook.

Instructor's note: *Divide the class into pairs. Each pair of students should complete the following tasks by referring to chapter 16 of the textbook.*

   A. Demonstrate trigger point and ice-and-stretch therapy to the upper trapezius, levator scapulae, sternocleidomastoid, scalenes, spleni, and posterior cervical muscles.

   B. Demonstrate soft-tissue mobilization to the thoracic and lumbar paraspinals, the quadratus lumborum, and the serratus posterior.

   C. Practice applying flexibility exercises to increase axial extension, cervical retraction, cervical flexion, and sternum extension.

   D. Practice applying flexibility exercises to the upper trapezius, scalene, and pectoralis muscles.

   E. Practice applying the following flexibility exercises:
   - Spinal twist
   - Quadratus lumborum stretch
   - Prolonged side-bending
   - Lumbar rock
   - Bent-over stretch
   - Knees-to-chest
   - Lateral trunk stretch
   - Thomas hip flexor stretch
   - Straight-leg raise
   - Piriformis stretch
   - Iliotibial band stretch
   - Lateral shift
   - Standing extension

2. For each of the following muscles or muscle groups, list appropriate exercises from among those just performed.

   A. Erector spinae

   B. Rectus femoris

C. Hamstrings

D. Hip external rotators

E. Internal and external obliques

F. Gluteus maximus

3. Practice maintaining a neutral lumbar spine.
4. Practice the following lumbar stabilization exercises:
   - Spine stabilization with arm movement
   - Spine stabilization with leg movement
   - Spine stabilization with arm and leg movement
   - Spine stabilization with arms and unsupported legs
   - Quadruped arm raise
   - Quadruped leg raise
   - Quadruped arm and leg raise
5. For the exercises just listed, at what point would you advance the athlete from single-limb to double-limb and combined upper- and lower-extremity exercises?

6. Practice the following cervical strengthening exercises:
   - Cervical isometrics
   - Prone neck retraction
   - Side-lying head lifts
   - Resisted cervical exercises
7. Practice the following upper back strengthening exercises:
   - Prone flys
   - Upright row
   - Upright press
   - Bouhler's
8. Practice the following lower back, abdominal, and pelvis exercises:
   - Posterior pelvic tilt
   - Trunk curl

- Crunch
- Oblique abdominal curl
- Supine leg exercises
- Side-lying sit-up
- Bridging
- Lateral trunk rotation
- Lunges
- Prone trunk extension
- Prone leg lift
- Latissimus pull-down

9. Practice the following agility and coordination exercises:
   - Resisted leg lifts
   - Ball exercises

10. Practice muscle energy techniques for the following lesions of the sacroiliac joint:
    - Anterior iliac subluxation: up-slip
    - Posterior iliac subluxation: up-slip
    - Sacral flexion
    - Forward torsion
    - Backward torsion
    - Anterior iliac rotation
    - Posterior iliac rotation
    - Pubic subluxation
    - Inflares and outflares

11. Use the case studies described in chapter 16 to apply a functional rehabilitation protocol for injuries to the trunk.

Instructor's note: *Following are a few of the case studies from chapter 16. Answers are included only for the ones presented here. The assignment of the remaining case studies is left to your discretion. You may also choose to create case studies of your own to further challenge your students.*

Case A. A javelin thrower injured his back last week in practice when he attempted to throw the javelin and felt a sudden pain in the right low back area. He presents to you stating that he applied ice to the injury when it occurred. The pain is now less than it was last week, but he still has pain when he rotates his trunk to the left and to the right. He has pain when he gets up from a chair and gets out of bed in the morning. His pain is worse at the end of the day. He has been taking it easy for a couple of days, but he is still unable to practice because of the pain. His pain is located in the right side of his low back area. He has no radiation of symptoms into the lower extremities, but he does get pain into the right buttock. When you examine him you find that he is unable to forward bend because of pain; side-bending to the left is too painful to perform, but side-bending to the right is better. Trunk rotation is more painful to the left than to the right. His spine has a lateral shift to the right in the lumbar region. Palpation reveals muscle spasm with tenderness in the right paraspinals and quadratus lumborum muscles. Pressure over the multifidi reproduces his buttock pain.

1. What is your first treatment?

2. Outline your treatment progression and indicate what guidelines you would use to advance him from one level to the next.

3. Give examples of specific exercises, including functional activities, prior to return to full participation.

Case B. A gymnast saw an orthopedic physician because of persistent complaints of low back pain that did not resolve after two weeks of reduced activity and modality treatments. The physician's diagnosis is a spondylolysis. A rehabilitation program is needed before she can return to competition.

Indicate the exercises you would avoid for this athlete, and outline a progression of exercises and activities that should be used in her therapeutic exercise program to return her to full participation.

Case C. A football lineman injured his back in a game four weeks ago. He was referred to an orthopedic surgeon because of continued low back and right lower-extremity pain. An MRI revealed that he has a disk bulge of 3 mm at L4-5. The physician indicates that he is not a surgical candidate because the problem may be resolved with rehabilitation, corticosteroid injections, or Medrol dose pack. He has had two of the three injections and reports significant relief of his back and leg pain. He is now coming to you for a rehabilitation program. He moves pretty well when he enters the examination room. He doesn't appear to hesitate to walk or to get up from a chair. You notice when he moves around the room, however, that he has very poor body mechanics, bending from the back to sit down and bending and twisting sideways to retrieve his backpack. His examination reveals a straight-leg raise to 50° on the right and 55° on the left, and his internal hip rotation is 20° bilaterally. In a forward bend, he is able to touch his fingers to his knees; in a side-bend he can touch just above his knee; and in backward bending he has good motion. Forward bending produces some discomfort. You notice that when he bends, most of the motion comes from the thoracic spine with the lumbar spine remaining essentially flat. The neurological examination reveals no deficiencies in sensory, motor, or reflex innervation. His gluteal muscles and abdominals are each tested at 4/5 strength. He is unable to perform a side sit-up on the right side. The paraspinals, quadratus lumborum, and hip external rotators are all tender to palpation, especially on the right, and you are able to palpate restriction of soft-tissue mobility in those tender areas. There is some restriction of joint mobility to PA tests in the lower lumbar spine.

1. What precautions would you have in treating this athlete?

2. What would your initial treatment program include?

3. List the techniques you would include in your first three treatment sessions.

4. Outline a progression of exercises you would use with this athlete and indicate what criteria you would have for progression from one level to the next in the program.

Case D. A 20-year-old wrestler reports that for the past week he has had trouble sleeping at night. He awakens with severe numbness and tingling in the right hand and a feeling of "pressure" in the forearm. The symptoms have been getting progressively worse since they started. He has some pain if he carries a lot of books between his classes, but feels OK when he is sitting in class. He doesn't recall having a specific injury. He has been wrestling for eight years and lifts weights in the preseason. His shoulder weight program includes bench press, military press, push-ups, flys, and biceps curls. Your examination confirms the doctor's diagnosis of thoracic outlet syndrome; although the Adson test is negative, you can reproduce his hand's tingling symptom when you perform a hyperextension maneuver. His posture is one of a forward-head and round-shoulder alignment. He has limited shoulder ROM in elevation and external rotation, and he is unable to move his elbow behind his shoulder in horizontal extension without discomfort in the chest. He has well-pronounced pectoralis and anterior deltoid muscles, but his rhomboids appear diminished and his rotator cuff muscles are weak.

1. What will be your instructions to this patient about posture?

2. What flexibility exercises will you give him, and what will be your guideline in determining when you begin them?

3. What are his strength deficiencies and muscle imbalances, and what exercises will you use to regain muscle balance?

LAB 19

Upper-Extremity Rehabilitation Protocol

The purpose of this lab is to provide you with case studies specific to upper-extremity rehabilitation.

Review material from chapters 17 through 19 of the textbook before completing this lab.

OBJECTIVES

- You should understand soft-tissue mobilization, joint mobilization, flexibility exericses, strengthening exercises, plyometrics, and functional activities for injuries to the shoulder, arm, elbow, wrist, hand, and fingers.

Name_____ Date_____

Activities

Use the case studies described in chapters 17 through 19 to apply a functional rehabilitation protocol for injuries to the shoulder, arm, elbow, wrist, hand, and fingers.

Instructor's note: *Following are a few of the case studies from chapters 17 through 19. Answers are included only for the ones presented here. The assignment of the remaining case studies is left to your discretion. You may also choose to create case studies of your own to further challenge your students.*

Case A. A 16-year-old basketball player was seen by the physician after suffering a right shoulder subluxation that occurred as he was going under the basket for a layup and his arm was caught and pulled into horizontal extension with external rotation. He has no history of prior injury. The physician has placed the arm in a sling and instructed you to begin a rehabilitation program for this athlete. It is one week since the injury. The athlete reports some difficulty sleeping at night because he can't get comfortable with the pain. He reports that he wears the sling all the time except while showering, as the physician has instructed him. On examination, you find some discoloration in the upper arm, but the swelling of last week is gone. There is some muscle spasm and tenderness to palpation of the infraspinatus, supraspinatus, teres minor, rhomboids, upper trapezius, and levator scapulae. You can notice atrophy of the supraspinatus already evident after one week. ROM of the shoulder is 40° flexion, 20° abduction, and −10° external rotation.

1. What will be your initial treatment?

2. Outline the exercises you will use during his first week of treatment.

3. What precautions must you take with his treatments?

4. Give a general outline of progression for this athlete's rehabilitation program, specifying what guidelines you will use to move from one level to the next.

Case B. A 40-year-old competitive tennis player reports to you that she has had shoulder pain during the last half of the tennis season. She is now unable to serve without pain. She has pain in the beginning of her warm-ups, but before a match begins the pain goes away. About 2 h after a match, her pain is significant. She has pain in the deltoid insertion area. The doctor has ruled out primary impingement but feels that a course of rehabilitation is necessary before the athlete returns to tennis. On examination she has full ROM except that she is lacking about 10° in elevation. Pain occurs in the end ranges of movement and above 90° of elevation. She has a forward-head, round-shoulder posture. Her glenohumeral rotators and abductors are weak and painful. She has weakness in the lower trapezius and rhomboids.

1. What is the cause of her secondary impingement?

2. What will you do to relieve the causes?

3. What will your first treatment include?

4. How will you advance her in her rehabilitation program?

5. What guidelines will you use for her progression?

6. What functional program will you use for her return to tennis?

Case C. An 18-year-old baseball pitcher underwent a glenohumeral capsular shift reconstruction one week ago because of instability. The surgeon wants you to begin the rehabilitation process today. The athlete's shoulder is in a bolster with the arm supported in partial abduction and internal rotation. Examination reveals a nicely healing surgical scar over the anterior-inferior aspect of the shoulder. Passive ROM measures 80° flexion, 80° abduction, and −10° external rotation. There is tenderness over the supraspinatus muscle belly, and the upper trapezius and levator scapulae muscles are tense and tender to palpation.

1. What will your treatment session today include?

2. Give this athlete an outline of your rehabilitation program, with an estimate of how long it will be before he begins a pitching program.

3. Outline his pitching progression program.

Case D. A 9-year-old baseball pitcher is in the middle of his season. For the past month he has experienced progressive medial elbow pain on his left throwing elbow. He is the team's top pitcher and usually pitches three days a week. An invitational tournament that his team is competing in is planned for next weekend, and he wants to pitch. His parents are reluctant to allow him to do so but want your opinion. He has full ROM of the elbow, but wrist extension is painful in the last 10°. Resisted pronation and wrist flexion are weak and painful. The medial epicondyle is tender to palpation and edematous.

1. What will be your recommendation to the athlete regarding the weekend invitational tournament?

2. What will be your recommendations on future pitching?

3. What treatment procedure will you recommend he follow to reduce the pain and inflammation?

4. What will be your instructions for exercises?

5. How much information will you give the athlete's parents?

Case E. A 30-year-old right-handed golfer injured his right elbow when he hit a divot and tore his ulnar collateral ligament. He attempted to continue playing through the season, but pain persisted. The elbow became unstable, and he underwent a medial collateral reconstruction. The surgery was 10 days ago, and he has been instructed by the surgeon to begin rehabilitation. The elbow is in a functional brace that is locked at −30° extension and 100° flexion. Supination is to neutral. Your examination reveals mild discoloration still present in the forearm and distal upper arm medially. There is spasm in the upper trapezius and biceps. Active ROM out of the brace is 60° extension to 100° flexion. Wrist extensors have 4/5 strength, the shoulder grossly has 4–/5 strength, the biceps and triceps are also 4–/5, and the wrist flexors are 3–/5. There are active trigger points in the forearm on the flexor and extensor surfaces.

1. What will be included in your first treatment session?

2. What precautions will you give the athlete?

3. When will you start pronation and supination motion activities?

4. What strengthening exercises will you include in the first week, and how will you advance them?

5. Where will you set the brace at week 5?

6. When will you start shoulder external rotation exercises?

7. What will be the functional exercise program you will establish for him, and when will you start it?

Case F. A 20-year-old right-handed gymnast fell off the balance beam five days ago, landing on a left hyperextended elbow and dislocating the elbow. It did not require surgery, but the orthopedist has placed the elbow in a 90° splint and wants you to begin rehabilitation on it today. Elbow ROM is –50° extension to 100° flexion. Supination is 10° and pronation is 20°. There is edema and ecchymosis surrounding the elbow and extending into the mid forearm and mid upper arm. Spasm is present in the biceps, triceps, and upper trapezius. Strength is difficult to test in the elbow, but the athlete complains of pain and offers minimal resistance to resisted elbow flexion and extension.

1. What will your first treatment session include?

2. What instructions for home exercises will you give the patient?

3. What exercises will you include as part of the first week's treatment program?

4. What are your goals for the first week?

5. What will be your progression of flexibility and strength exercises?

6. What functional exercise program will you include for rehabilitation?

Case G. A 21-year-old hockey forward suffered a fracture of the neck of the fourth MCP when he was involved in a fight during a game and hit an opponent. The hand was casted for two weeks and then placed in a splint that can be removed for his rehabilitation activities. The fracture is stable, so the physician wants to wean him from the splint over the next two weeks. The initial examination reveals some swelling in the hand and fingers. Wrist flexion is 50° and wrist extension is 65°. Ulnar deviation and radial deviation are 10°. Supination is 70° and pronation is 90°. MCP flexion is 45°, PIP flexion is 80°, and DIP flexion is 60°. He is unable to make a complete fist. The MCP and IP joints can extend passively to 0°. He is unable to simultaneously flex the MCP and extend the IP joints.

1. What do you suspect his primary problems to be?

2. What will be included in your first three treatment sessions with him, assuming no regression with your treatments?

3. What will your initial goals during the first week be for him?

4. What precautions must you be aware of in treating him?

5. Describe three home exercises you will give him at the time of your first treatment.

6. List four strengthening exercises you will use with this patient.

7. What functional exercises will you incorporate into his rehabilitation program before he returns to hockey?

Case H. A 16-year-old right-handed volleyball setter suffered a dislocated dominant middle finger three weeks ago. The finger has been in a partial flexion splint for the past three weeks. The physician has instructed her to tape the finger to her ring finger throughout the day except when in rehabilitation. She has been moving the wrist and MCP joint, but the finger has been immobilized since the injury. The edema is gone, but the finger is stiff in the IP joints. Passive DIP extension/flexion is −15°/30°, and the PIP extension/flexion is −30°/50°. Active DIP extension/flexion is −20°/25°, and the PIP extension/flexion is −40°/50°. She is unable to make a complete fist because the middle finger does not flex into the palm. Her grip strength measurement is 13.6 kg (30 lb) on the right and 31.8 kg (70 lb) on the left. There is tenderness over the PIP collateral ligaments, especially on the radial side.

1. What will your first treatment goals be for her today?

2. What will you attempt to accomplish in the next three treatments?

3. How will you accomplish those goals?

4. What precautions should you consider in her treatments?

5. What are two exercises you will send home with her today?

6. What strengthening exercises will you use?

7. What functional activities will you eventually include in her therapeutic exercise program?

Case I. A 24-year-old crew team member underwent a surgical release of his right nondominant first dorsal compartment two days ago. He has just seen the physician, who has removed the surgical dressing and instructed him to begin exercising the wrist and thumb. The athlete has a splint to wear throughout the day except for treatments. There is some swelling and tenderness over the scar. The wrist has good motion, but the thumb moves 10° at the MCP joint and 30° at the IP joint. There is some tenderness to radial deviation, but motion is full.

1. Explain what your treatment today will include.

2. What instructions will you give him for home treatment?

3. What precautions must be considered?

4. What kind of ROM exercises will you give him?

5. When will you start working on strength, and what will the first strengthening exercises include?

6. What functional exercises will you advance him to before he returns to competition?

LAB 20

Lower-Extremity Rehabilitation Protocol

The purpose of this lab is to provide you with case studies specific to lower-extremity rehabilitation.

Review material from chapters 20 through 22 of the textbook before completing this lab.

OBJECTIVES

- You should understand soft-tissue mobilization, joint mobilization, flexibility exercises, strengthening exercises, proprioception exercises, and functional activities for injuries to the foot, ankle, lower leg, knee, thigh, and hip.

Name_____   Date_____

Activities

Use the case studies described in chapters 20 through 22 to apply a functional rehabilitation protocol for injuries to the foot, ankle, lower leg, knee, thigh, and hip.

Case A. A 16-year-old volleyball hitter jumped up for a hit and landed on another player's foot three days ago, causing an inversion sprain to the right ankle. She felt a pop and had immediate swelling at the time of the injury. She was unable to bear weight on the foot at the time. X rays were negative, but she was placed on crutches, weight bearing to tolerance. She has used ice, elevation, and taping periodically for the past three days but comes to you today to start her rehabilitation program. She denies any previous ankle injury. So far she has performed only alphabet exercises because all other activities cause too much pain. She can put about 11.3 kg (25 lb) of weight on the foot before complaining of pain in the lateral ankle and above the ankle joint. Her pain is located over the anterior talofibular, anterior tibiofibular, and calcaneofibular joints with most of the pain over the first two ligaments. She has moderate swelling of the ankle, foot, and toes with ecchymosis over the midfoot to the toes. She is able to wiggle her toes about 50% normally. Her ankle ROM is −10° dorsiflexion with pain, 45° plantar flexion, 10° inversion with pain, and 10° eversion. Her ankle strength is restricted by pain on dorsiflexion and inversion. She is unable to bear weight on the foot for assessment of antigravity strength of the calf, but you are easily able to manually resist plantar flexion. Eversion is 4/5. Joint mobility is normal. Soft-tissue mobility is limited by the edema present, but you are unable to palpate any abnormal soft-tissue restriction.

1. What are your goals with today's treatment?

2. What treatment will you provide for her today?

3. What home instructions will you give her?

4. What precautions will you give her?

5. What will be your guidelines for when she can begin resistive weight-bearing exercises?

6. When she is able, list three agility exercises you will include in her program.

7. What will your functional testing include prior to her return to full sport participation?

Case B. A 16-year-old female cross country runner fractured her right tibia in a motor vehicle accident five years ago. The leg was casted at that time for two months before she underwent a rehabilitation program. One month ago she was competing in a cross country race and began experiencing right shin and foot numbness and burning. Since then she has experienced the same symptoms during her workouts. She underwent an anterior and a posterior compartment release and removal of extensive scar tissue two weeks ago. The surgeon wants her to begin rehabilitation today. She is partial weight bearing on crutches, but the surgeon has instructed her to ambulate without the crutches in the next couple of days. She admits that she lacks the confidence to do without the crutches. Your assessment reveals well-healed surgical scars anteriorly and posteriorly on the lower leg. Mild edema is present; there is stiffness to passive ROM but no pain. Dorsiflexion is –5°, and plantar flexion is 35°. Inversion and eversion are 30°. Palpation reveals mild soft-tissue restriction around the surgical scars and moderate tissue restriction in the calf and anterior lower leg.

1. What are your goals for her first treatment with you today?

2. What, if any, modalities will you use and why?

3. What exercises will you initiate today?

4. What home program and instructions will you give to her before she leaves today?

5. What are your goals for her for the next two weeks, and how will you attempt to accomplish them?

6. What specific activities will you have her perform the first day she is on a treadmill?

7. Outline a progressive running program that you will give her when she is ready to begin running.

Case C. A 16-year-old wrestler suffered a left ankle lateral malleolar fracture during a wrestling match. The athlete underwent an ORIF the following day and was placed on crutches, non-weight bearing for two weeks; he then advanced to partial weight bearing. He is now four weeks postoperative and is not yet full weight bearing, although the surgeon has instructed him to begin weight bearing to tolerance and advance to weight bearing without the crutches. He admits to you that he is apprehensive about putting weight on the leg for fear of breaking it again. The lower leg was in a cast following surgery until yesterday, when the cast was removed. On examination, his ankle has −10° dorsiflexion, 30° plantar flexion, 0° eversion, and 5° inversion. Ankle strength in these directions is 2+/5 in the available ranges of motion. His hip and knee ROM are normal, but strength of all the muscle groups is 4–/5. The surgical scar is well healed, but there is sloughing skin around the ankle and there are dry scabs over the wound. Palpation reveals stiffness of soft tissue around the ankle and into the foot. The foot is mildly enlarged, but there is no pitting edema. Joint mobility of the ankle joints is restricted to no more than 30% normal, and the intertarsal and metatarsal joints are restricted to 50% normal mobility.

1. What are your goals for today's treatment session?

2. What home program will you send with him today?

3. The athlete wants to attend a wrestling camp that is scheduled for 10 weeks from now; what do you tell him when he asks if he will be able to attend the camp?

4. List your long- and short-term goals for him for the next six weeks.

5. What will be your criteria for advancing him to closed kinetic chain exercises?

6. List three closed kinetic exercises that you will give him the first day these are in his program.

7. List three non-weight-bearing exercises you will give him in the next week.

8. List three agility exercises you will use in his program, as well as criteria that he must pass before they are used.

Case D. A 17-year-old male gymnast suffered a grade II sprain of his right medial collateral ligament on a rings dismount three days ago. The physician wants him started on a rehabilitation program. For the past three days he has used ice, elevation, compression, and electrical stimulation for edema control. He is on crutches with a hinged brace set at 0° and 90°. He is bearing about 75% of his body weight on the right leg when he ambulates. There is moderate swelling with tenderness to palpation along the medial collateral ligament. Both his hip and hamstring strength are grossly 4/5. He has an extensor lag of 15°. He reports mild pain unless he attempts to bend the knee past 60°; the pain then becomes moderate. Patellar mobility is normal.

1. What will your first treatment for him today include?

2. What home program will you give him before he leaves your facility today?

3. Outline the exercise program you will have him perform for the next week.

4. How will you determine his progression?

5. List three open kinetic chain and three closed kinetic chain exercises you will have him perform within the next two weeks, and list them in the order in which you will give them to him.

6. What agility exercises will you include in his program?

7. What plyometric exercises will you use?

8. Describe the functional activities you will use in your assessment to determine when he is ready to return to full sport participation.

Case E. A 16-year-old female cross country runner has had left knee pain for the past month. The pain has progressed so that it now interferes with her workouts and continues during walking. The physician has diagnosed her with anterior knee pain and wants her to begin rehabilitation. Your examination reveals genu valgus and recurvatum with foot pronation in standing. Her running shoes have excessive wear on the lateral posterior heel so that the midsole is evident. The shoes have a sewn curved last. Her rearfoot and forefoot have excessive mobility. Straight-leg raise is to 70°; ankle dorsiflexion in rearfoot neutral is 0°. She has a positive Ober's test, and deep palpation reveals tenderness along the distal iliotibial band. Her quadriceps strength is 4–/5, lower abdominal strength 3/5, and hip extension strength 4/5. Patellar alignment assessment reveals a posterior and lateral tilt. Patellar tracking in long sitting is lateral. In standing, lateral patellar tracking is less. During performance of a step-down exercise, pain is produced, and the knee wobbles with minimal activity apparent. Palpation of the posterior patellar surface reveals tenderness medially and laterally, especially over the inferior aspect.

1. What will your treatment for her today include?

2. What instructions will you send her home with today?

3. What will you tell her when she asks what she should do about her workouts?

4. Given her signs, what part of the ROM would you expect her to have the most pain in?

5. List two elements you will use to strengthen the VMO during the first week.

6. What are your short-term and long-term goals for her, and when do you expect her to achieve them?

Case F. One week ago, a 30-year-old male tennis player was sprinting to return a ball at the net when he felt a tear in his right hamstring. He was unable to walk and sought medical attention. The physician has diagnosed a grade II hamstring strain and wants him to begin rehabilitation. The athlete ambulates with a slight antalgic gait. His knee motion is 115° flexion to −15° extension. Left straight-leg raise is 60°, but the patient states that he has always been tight in his hamstrings. His hamstring strength is 3/5 and painful to attempts at resistance. His quadriceps, ankle, and hip strength are grossly 4/5. There is a large area of ecchymosis that runs on the posterior leg from the proximal thigh below the gluteal fold to about 10 cm (3.9 in.) distal to the knee. The ecchymotic region is most tender in the darkest discoloration area along the posterolateral thigh. There is a small indentation with tenderness to palpation about 10 cm distal and 10 cm lateral to the ischial tuberosity.

1. What will you include in today's treatment for him?

2. What home program will you give him before he leaves today?

3. What are your short-term goals for him and when do you expect to achieve them?

4. Outline the course of exercises for him for the next two weeks.

5. What functional activities will you include in his program?

6. What will your criteria be for permitting him to return to full sport participation?

Case G. A 25-year-old distance runner presents with complaints of right buttock and posterior thigh pain that has become progressively worse for the past three weeks. He has recently increased his distance from 6.4 to 9.7 km (4 to 6 miles). The pain occurs about 4.8 km (3 miles) into his run and stays there. He reports that when he gets up from his desk after sitting for about 45 min, his right buttock is painful until he walks around for a few minutes. He had a back injury about five years ago that was treated, and he hasn't had any problems since then. Standing trunk motions do not elicit pain in any direction. When he lies supine on the treatment table, his right leg is externally rotated about 20° more than his left. Placing the hip in 60° flexion, adduction, and internal rotation elicits pain in the right buttock. Straight-leg raising is to 70° and negative for sciatic pain. Palpating the right buttock with the athlete in prone reveals tenderness in the midbuttock region to deep pressure. You can feel a tightness in the muscle in this region. Resisted hip external rotation in this position is painful. Hip rotation is weak.

1. What other tests should you perform to eliminate any other possible cause of his problem?

2. What do you suspect he has?

3. What will be your first treatment for him today?

4. What instructions for home treatments will you give him before he leaves today?

5. What will your goals for the first week of treatment include?

6. What will you tell him when he asks you if he can continue running?

Case H. A 16-year-old sprinter injured her left hip when she was practicing three days ago. She has continual pain in the proximal inner thigh with some discoloration along the middle aspect of the inner thigh. She is unable to walk normally because of the pain. Your examination reveals hip abduction to 20°, limited by pain. She is unable to lift the leg against gravity into adduction. Hip flexion is 4/5 but not as tender as adduction. The inner thigh area feels tight and is tender to palpation from the middle thigh to the groin.

1. What do you suspect is her injury?

2. What other differential tests will you perform?

3. What will her treatment today include?

4. What instructions for home care will you give her today?

5. Outline the progression of therapeutic exercises you will provide her.

6. What modalities will you use with her and why?

Case I. A 17-year-old female forward soccer player reports that she has had progressive anterior hip pain for the past four weeks. It is to the point that it bothers her on stairs and in walking and standing. She ambulates with an antalgic gait, using a shortened stride length and keeping the hip flexed and in a forward trunk lean. Your examination reveals tenderness to resisted hip flexion that increases with resisted knee extension applied simultaneously. Hip flexion is weak. Passive stretch of prone hip extension with knee flexion is more uncomfortable than hip extension with the knee extended. There is tenderness to palpation of the AIIS, and pressure on this area reproduces her pain.

1. What do you suspect her problem is?

2. What other differential diagnoses should you eliminate and how would you do this?

3. Explain what your treatment for her today will include.

4. What home instructions will you give her before she leaves today?

5. Outline the rehabilitation program you will place her on over the next two weeks.

6. How will you determine when she is ready to resume full sport participation?

ABOUT THE AUTHORS

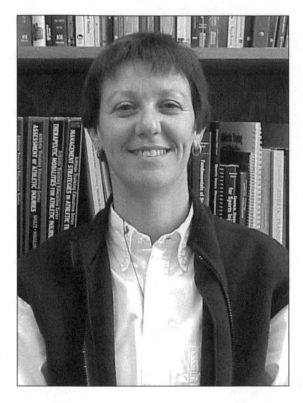

Linda S. Levy, MEd, is an instructor and athletic trainer at Plymouth State College in Plymouth, New Hampshire. She has served as an athletic trainer for 22 years and has taught rehabilitation and therapeutic exercise for 8 years. She is a member of the National Athletic Trainers' Association (NATA).

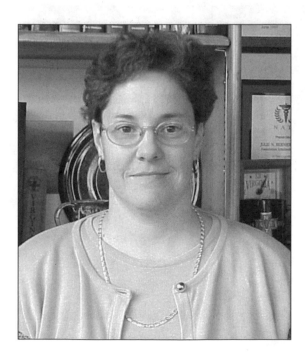

Julie N. Bernier, EdD, ATC, has been the athletic training program director at Plymouth State College in Plymouth, New Hampshire, since 1990. She serves on the editorial board of the *Journal of Athletic Training,* and is vice chair of grants for the research committee of the NATA Research and Education Foundation (NATA-REF). Dr. Bernier is a member of the NATA and the American College of Sports Medicine.

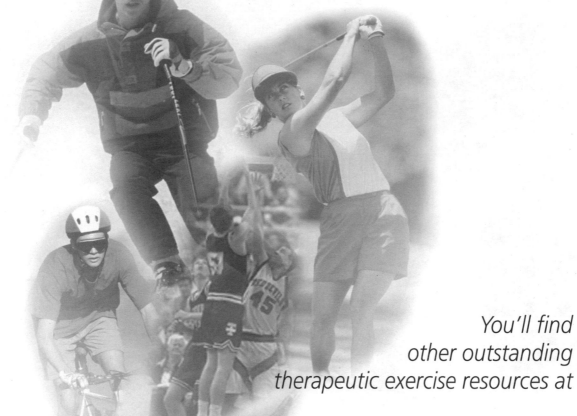